LUTEIN AND ZEAXANTHIN FOR BEGINNERS

Eye-Catching Insights, Navigating Lutein And Zeaxanthin For Optimal Vision, Discover The Power Of Natural Eye Nutrients For Long-Term Health

Georgette Lockett

DISCLAIMER

The author of this book is not affiliated, associated, endorsed, sponsored, or approved by any company or individual. The views and opinions expressed in this book are solely those of the author and do not necessarily reflect the official policy or position of any entity.

The author hereby disclaims any relationship, collaboration, or partnership with any company or individual mentioned in this book. Any references to products, services, or individuals are provided for informational purposes only and should not be construed as an endorsement or recommendation.

Readers are advised to exercise their own judgment and discretion when applying the information provided in this book. The author shall not be held responsible for any actions taken by readers based on the content of this book.

This book is intended for general informational purposes only, and the author makes no representations or warranties of any kind, express or implied, about the completeness, accuracy, reliability, suitability, or availability of the information contained herein. Any reliance on the information in this book is at the reader's own risk.

The author reserves the right to update, change, or modify any information in this book without notice. It is the responsibility of the reader to verify any information before taking any actions based on the content of this book.

By reading this book, the reader acknowledges and agrees to the terms of this disclaimer.

INTRODUCTION

Overview Of Lutein And Zeaxanthin

Lutein and Zeaxanthin are naturally occurring xanthophyll carotenoids that play an important role in maintaining normal eye health. These chemicals, which are present in a variety of fruits and vegetables, help greatly to the preservation of eyesight and general well-being. The purpose of this book is to dive into the significance of Lutein and Zeaxanthin, investigating their dietary sources, absorption methods, and biological roles inside the human body.

Importance Of Lutein And Zeaxanthin For Eye Health

The eyes are very vulnerable to oxidative stress and damage produced by sunlight and environmental factors. Lutein and Zeaxanthin are natural antioxidants that accumulate in the retina and create the macular pigment. This pigment acts as a barrier, absorbing high-energy blue light and neutralizing free radicals, avoiding oxidative damage to the retina's sensitive cells. Lutein and Zeaxanthin are linked to a lower risk of age-related macular degeneration (AMD), a frequent cause of visual loss in older persons.

Dietary Sources And Absorption

While the human body cannot produce Lutein and Zeaxanthin, they are plentiful in a variety of fruits and vegetables. These carotenoids are abundant in leafy greens such as kale, spinach, and collard greens, as well as other foods such as maize and eggs. Because lutein and zeaxanthin are fat-soluble molecules, their absorption is enhanced when eaten with dietary fats. Incorporating these items into a well-balanced diet increases the bioavailability of these critical nutrients, promoting absorption and use inside the body.

Biological Functions In The Human Body

Lutein and Zeaxanthin have a variety of biological roles apart from their significance in eye health. According to research, they may have a role in boosting skin health, supporting cognitive function, and even contributing to cardiovascular health. They help to reduce inflammation and fight oxidative stress throughout the body as antioxidants. These carotenoids, with their many roles, highlight the interdependence of nutrition and general health.

We will look at each aspect of Lutein and Zeaxanthin in this book, from their responsibilities in eye health to their larger benefits to general well-being. Understanding the significance of including these chemicals in a well-balanced diet is critical for supporting long-term health and avoiding age-related disorders.

The following chapters will dig further into the complicated world of Lutein and Zeaxanthin, exploring their distinct advantages, possible concerns of insufficiency, and practical measures to ensure appropriate intake. Readers will have a thorough knowledge of how Lutein and Zeaxanthin contribute to a holistic approach to health and well-being by the conclusion of this book.

CHAPTER 1

Basics Of Lutein And Zeaxanthin

Lutein and zeaxanthin are two carotenoids that are highly valued for their critical functions in supporting excellent eye health and general wellness. Understanding their chemical structure and characteristics reveals information about their amazing activities inside the human body.

Chemical Structure And Properties

Lutein and zeaxanthin are carotenoids from the xanthophyll subgroup, which are pigment molecules produced by plants. They have different structural traits defined by their molecular formula and carbon atom arrangement, which contribute to their specific properties.

1. **Lutein Structure:** Lutein is made up of 40 carbon atoms and two oxygen molecules, resulting in a polyene chain, which is a molecule with lengthy

chains and alternating single and double bonds. Its structure enables it to absorb blue light wavelengths, functioning as a natural filter against dangerous high-energy light such as ultraviolet (UV) rays and protecting the retina.

2. **Zeaxanthin Structure:** Similar to lutein, zeaxanthin has 40 carbon atoms and two oxygen molecules. It does, however, have a somewhat different configuration, which influences its location in the eye. It is abundant in the central macula, where it improves visual acuity and protects against oxidative damage.

Natural Occurrence In Foods

Both lutein and zeaxanthin may be found in a variety of fruits and vegetables, especially those with brilliant hues such as green leafy vegetables (kale, spinach), yellow-orange food (corn, squash), and egg yolks. These molecules contribute to the color of these meals while also acting as antioxidants.

Comparison With Other Carotenoids

Although lutein and zeaxanthin are related to other carotenoids such as beta-carotene and astaxanthin, their activities and locations in the body vary greatly.

• **Beta-carotene:** Unlike lutein and zeaxanthin, which are primarily found in the eyes, beta-carotene is turned into vitamin A and has a variety of functions in eyesight, skin health, and immunological function.

• **Astaxanthin:** This carotenoid is known for its significant antioxidant qualities, which assist in cardiovascular health, skin protection, and oxidative stress reduction.

What distinguishes lutein and zeaxanthin is their localized concentration in the macular area of the retina, where they act as structural components of the eye.

These carotenoids are critical in protecting the eyes from oxidative stress caused by blue light exposure and other environmental variables. Their presence in the retina aids in the maintenance of visual acuity, the prevention of age-related macular degeneration (AMD), and the general health of the eye.

Understanding lutein and zeaxanthin's molecular structures, natural sources, and different functions lays the groundwork for comprehending their importance in improving eye health and general well-being.

CHAPTER 2

Role In Eye Health

Two essential carotenoids contained in the human eye, lutein, and zeaxanthin, play critical roles in maintaining good visual function and protecting against eye disorders.

Macular Pigment And Its Significance

The macula, a tiny portion of the retina near the center, is in charge of detailed central vision. The principal components of the macular pigment are lutein and zeaxanthin, which create a protective layer that functions as a natural blue light filter. This pigment absorbs high-energy light wavelengths, especially blue light, protecting the underlying retinal tissues from oxidative stress damage.

Protection Against Age-Related Macular Degeneration (Amd)

A common cause of visual loss in the elderly is age-related macular degeneration (AMD). The antioxidant capabilities of lutein and zeaxanthin are critical in countering oxidative stress, which contributes to the formation and progression of AMD. These carotenoids may help minimize the risk and delay the progression of AMD, especially the dry variety, by neutralizing free radicals and lowering inflammation in the retina.

Relationship With Visual Performance

Lutein and zeaxanthin have been linked to improved visual performance in addition to reducing eye disorders. Their presence in macular pigment affects a variety of visual processes, including contrast sensitivity and glare tolerance. According to research, those with greater levels of these carotenoids may have superior visual acuity and adaptability to diverse light settings, which contributes to overall visual comfort and clarity.

Understanding the importance of Lutein and Zeaxanthin in eye health highlights the need to include these carotenoids in one's diet. While these chemicals cannot be produced by the human body, their abundance in specific foods provides an opportunity for people to support their ocular health via dietary choices.

Individuals may increase their intake of these important carotenoids by adding foods high in Lutein and Zeaxanthin, such as leafy green vegetables (spinach, kale), maize, eggs, and orange/yellow fruits and vegetables. Supplements are also available for people looking to enhance their levels, particularly if their food consumption is inadequate.

In conclusion, as components of the macular pigment, lutein, and zeaxanthin play an important role in maintaining eye health. Their capacity to combat oxidative stress and support visual functioning emphasizes the relevance of carotenoids in preserving healthy vision and preventing age-related eye disorders. Including them in one's diet is a proactive step toward supporting long-term eye health and visual well-being.

CHAPTER 3

Absorption And Bioavailability

Two vital carotenoids, lutein and zeaxanthin, play critical roles in maintaining good eye health. Understanding how these substances are absorbed and their bioavailability is critical for getting the most out of them.

Absorption Mechanisms In The Body

The small intestine is where lutein and zeaxanthin are absorbed. These carotenoids are fat-soluble, which means they need dietary fat to be absorbed. The process includes the incorporation of lutein and zeaxanthin into mixed micelles with bile salts and other lipids. This enables carotenoids to pass through the hydrophobic environment of the gut mucosa.

Once absorbed, lutein and zeaxanthin are carried in the lymphatic system by chylomicrons, which are lipoprotein particles and finally reach the circulation. These carotenoids are then distributed to numerous tissues, including the eyes, where they provide protection.

Factors Influencing Bioavailability

Several variables impact lutein and zeaxanthin bioavailability. As previously stated, the presence of dietary fats improves absorption. However, the matrix in which these carotenoids exist is equally important. The bioavailability of lutein and zeaxanthin from fruits and vegetables, for example, may vary depending on their cellular structure and the presence of other nutrients.

Cooking procedures may influence bioavailability. Heat treatment, such as steaming or boiling, may break down cell walls, making lutein and zeaxanthin more absorbable.

Furthermore, the ingestion of certain meals, such as those high in fat, may increase carotenoid absorption.

Supplements Vs. Natural Sources

While lutein and zeaxanthin pills are available, it is typically suggested that these carotenoids be obtained from natural dietary sources. Whole foods include a complex matrix of nutrients and substances that may work together to improve absorption and utilization.

Furthermore, carotenoid absorption via supplements may vary from that of naturally occurring sources. Other carotenoids and phytochemicals included in meals may lead to a more balanced and efficient absorption.

A diversified intake of carotenoids is ensured by including a range of colored fruits and vegetables in the diet. Lutein and zeaxanthin are abundant in leafy greens, broccoli, peas, and egg yolks.

Adopting a diet high in these foods benefits not only your eyes but also your general health.

Understanding the absorption processes and variables affecting lutein and zeaxanthin bioavailability allows people to make more educated dietary choices. Achieving a mix of natural dietary sources and, if required, supplementation may help optimize carotenoid levels, encouraging long-term eye health and general vigor.

CHAPTER 4

Health Benefits Beyond Vision

Certainly, lutein and zeaxanthin stand out among the essential nutrients for eye health. However, their advantages extend well beyond visual assistance.

Antioxidant Properties

Lutein and zeaxanthin, which are well-known for their presence in the eyes, are potent antioxidants. They function as "ocular antioxidants," protecting the eyes from dangerous high-energy light and free radicals, lowering the incidence of AMD and cataracts. Their involvement in protecting the eyes from oxidative stress extends to other physiological systems as well.

Cardiovascular Health

These carotenoids go beyond ocular advantages by favorably influencing cardiovascular health. Their antioxidant properties help to reduce oxidative stress by avoiding cholesterol oxidation, which is a critical stage in the development of arterial plaques. According to research, consuming more lutein and zeaxanthin may help lower the risk of cardiovascular disease.

Skin Health

Lutein and zeaxanthin may be more than just eye-savers; they may also be skin-savers. They fight free radicals caused by UV exposure as antioxidants, possibly minimizing skin damage and premature aging. Incorporating these carotenoids into your diet or taking supplements may help protect your skin from oxidative stress and keep it healthy and supple.

Understanding their significance in providing protection other than eyesight emphasizes the need to include these nutrients in our everyday diet.

Absorption Mechanisms in the Body: Lutein and zeaxanthin are absorbed in the small intestine, which is aided by dietary lipids and bile acids. Combining these carotenoids with a source of healthy fats improves absorption, making them more accessible for the body to use efficiently.

Factors Influencing Bioavailability: The presence of dietary lipids, individual differences in metabolism, and food processing processes all influence lutein and zeaxanthin absorption. They may be better absorbed if consumed with fat-rich meals or with a balanced diet.

Supplements vs. Natural Sources: While supplements are convenient, obtaining lutein and zeaxanthin from natural sources such as leafy green vegetables (spinach, kale), eggs, and certain fruits (kiwi, grapes) ensures a variety of nutrients and compounds that may enhance absorption and effectiveness.

In essence, acknowledging the many advantages of lutein and zeaxanthin emphasizes their importance beyond eye health. Incorporating these carotenoids into daily meals not only benefits eyesight but also general well-being, demonstrating their holistic health effect.

CHAPTER 5

Recommended Dietary Intake And Deficiency

Recommended Daily Allowance (RDA)

Official health organizations do not specify the recommended dietary intake for lutein and zeaxanthin. However, evidence shows that ingesting 6-20 mg of these carotenoids each day may provide considerable health advantages. These levels are often attained by eating a diet high in fruits and vegetables.

Symptoms Of Deficiency

While no distinct deficiency condition for Lutein and Zeaxanthin has been found, their scarcity in the diet may influence eye health. Inadequate consumption may raise risk factors for age-related macular degeneration (AMD) and cataracts.

Because of decreased amounts of these carotenoids, AMD is linked with diminished macular pigment density.

Groups At Risk

Certain groups may be particularly vulnerable to Lutein and Zeaxanthin deficiency:

1. **Elderly individuals:** Age-related macular degeneration becomes more common as individuals age, and a lack of these carotenoids in the diet may worsen the risk.

2. **Individuals Who Make Poor Dietary Choices:** People who eat a diet low in fruits and vegetables may not receive enough Lutein and Zeaxanthin.

3. **Smokers:** Cigarette smoke depletes antioxidants in the body, particularly Lutein and Zeaxanthin, placing smokers at a greater risk of deficiency.

4. **Individuals with Malabsorption Issues:** Certain digestive problems or surgical procedures that alter

nutrient absorption may result in decreased amounts of these carotenoids being absorbed from the diet.

Deficiency Correction and Adequate Intake

To counteract any inadequacies, a well-balanced diet rich in Lutein and Zeaxanthin sources should be prioritized. Leafy greens like spinach and kale, as well as yellow and orange vegetables like maize and squash, and eggs, are good sources.

Supplements may be considered in circumstances when food consumption is inadequate. However, before supplementing, speak with a healthcare practitioner since excessive quantities might have negative side effects or interact with specific drugs.

It is critical to raise awareness among healthcare practitioners and the general public about the role of these carotenoids in eye health. Promoting dietary recommendations that promote the intake of foods rich in Lutein and Zeaxanthin may considerably reduce the risk of eye-related disorders caused by their lack.

CHAPTER 6

Lutein And Zeaxanthin In Foods

Two potent carotenoids, lutein, and zeaxanthin, are essential for maintaining good eye health. While supplementation is an option, getting these nutrients from natural food sources is typically a more preferable and balanced strategy.

Rich Food Sources

Several fruits and vegetables stand out as high-quality sources of lutein and zeaxanthin. These carotenoids are prevalent in leafy greens such as kale, spinach, and collard greens. Other vegetables, such as peas and broccoli, add to a lutein and zeaxanthin-rich diet. Furthermore, some fruits, such as kiwi and grapes, contain significant levels of these chemicals.

Cooking And Processing Effects On Content

Understanding the effects of cooking and food processing on lutein and zeaxanthin content is critical for retaining their nutritional advantages. These carotenoids are heat-sensitive and may be destroyed in part during cooking. However, as compared to boiling, other cooking techniques, such as steaming or microwaving, are less harmful to the level of these chemicals. Additionally, using healthy fats in cooking, such as olive oil, may improve lutein and zeaxanthin absorption.

Dietary Strategies To Increase Intake

Individuals may use a variety of dietary techniques to increase their intake of lutein and zeaxanthin. Incorporating a variety of colored fruits and vegetables into daily meals guarantees a wide range of carotenoids, including lutein and zeaxanthin.

Smoothies, salads, and stir-fries are easy ways to blend various carotenoid-rich foods. Furthermore, being attentive to cooking techniques and avoiding excessive food processing might aid in preserving the nutritional content of these chemicals.

It is crucial to remember that lutein and zeaxanthin interact along with other nutrients to maintain general eye health, including vitamins C and E, zinc, and omega-3 fatty acids. As a result, eating a well-balanced, nutrient-dense diet benefits not just the health of the eyes but also the general well-being of the body.

Finally, Chapter 6 highlights the need to get lutein and zeaxanthin from natural dietary sources. Individuals may increase their intake of these critical carotenoids by including a range of colored fruits and vegetables in daily meals and being attentive to cooking techniques, encouraging not just optimum eye health but also overall nutritional well-being.

CHAPTER 7

Supplementation And Safety

Lutein and zeaxanthin supplementation has gained popularity owing to its important functions in eye health and general well-being. Understanding the many types of supplements, their quantities, and safety concerns is critical for anyone looking to supplement their consumption beyond food sources.

Supplement Forms And Dosages

Lutein and zeaxanthin supplements are available in a variety of formats, including capsules, pills, and soft gels. Their daily doses typically range from 6 to 20 milligrams (mg), with lutein and zeaxanthin combos being particularly prevalent. However, a healthcare practitioner should be consulted to establish the optimal dose depending on individual requirements.

Potential Side Effects And Interactions

When used in the prescribed quantities, lutein and zeaxanthin supplements are generally regarded as safe for most people. Excessive consumption, on the other hand, may result in carotenodermia, a harmless disorder that causes the skin to become somewhat yellowish. There may also be interactions with some drugs, notably those that impact blood thinning or cholesterol levels. It is best to see a healthcare practitioner before beginning any supplement program, particularly if you have a medical condition or are using medication.

Safety Considerations

The safety profile of lutein and zeaxanthin derived from food is well known. However, while choosing supplements, it is essential to ensure their quality, purity, and adherence to production requirements. Checking for third-party certifications or reputed companies might aid in the selection of dependable supplements.

Understanding how carotenoids interact with other nutrients, particularly in a balanced diet, is critical. Supplements may be useful, but they should not be used instead of a balanced diet rich in fruits, vegetables, and other nutrient-dense foods.

Furthermore, pregnant or nursing women should proceed with care and seek medical counsel before beginning any supplemental plan. A varied diet rich in fruits and vegetables may naturally boost the consumption of these carotenoids.

Although uncommon, it is also vital to be wary of any allergic responses. Individuals who are sensitive to marigolds, maize, or other comparable compounds may be allergic to supplements containing lutein and zeaxanthin produced from these sources.

In conclusion, although lutein and zeaxanthin supplements may be beneficial, particularly for people with restricted dietary access or specific health issues, they are not a replacement for a well-balanced diet. Getting these nutrients from a variety of meals is still the most sustainable and recommended technique for the majority of people. When considering supplements, careful consideration of dose, quality, and individual health circumstances assures safe and effective usage, contributing favorably to overall health and ocular well-being.

CHAPTER 8

Research And Scientific Studies

Because of their various biological characteristics, lutein and zeaxanthin have been the topic of much scientific research. Understanding their involvement in human health has been a focus of study, with numerous advantages and uses revealed.

Notable Research Findings

Lutein and zeaxanthin have long been recognized as powerful antioxidants, according to research. These carotenoids are thought to defend against oxidative stress, which is linked to a variety of chronic disorders. Furthermore, their buildup in the macula of the eye implies a major contribution to visual health, notably in lowering the incidence of AMD and cataracts.

Furthermore, studies have been conducted to investigate the relationship between lutein and zeaxanthin consumption and cognitive performance. Some research suggests that these carotenoids may improve cognitive ability and memory, but further research is needed.

Ongoing Studies And Areas Of Interest

Continuous research is being conducted to better understand the processes by which lutein and zeaxanthin exert their effects. To maximize their health advantages, researchers are investigating their bioavailability, transport, and metabolism inside the body.

Another area of active research is the possible cardiovascular advantages of lutein and zeaxanthin. Early research suggests a relationship between these carotenoids and cardiovascular health, perhaps lowering the risk of heart disease. Further study is being conducted to explain these pathways.

Controversies And Debates

Despite multiple research supporting the advantages of lutein and zeaxanthin, there is still disagreement about their intake. Some suggest that getting these carotenoids from natural dietary sources is preferable because of possible synergistic effects with other nutrients found in whole foods. There is continuous debate concerning the effectiveness of supplements vs whole foods in providing the intended health advantages.

Furthermore, there are disagreements about recommended doses for various groups and the possible hazards associated with excessive consumption, even though adverse effects from natural food sources are exceedingly uncommon.

As our knowledge of lutein and zeaxanthin grows, current research strives to uncover their full potential and prospective uses in the prevention of chronic illnesses and the promotion of general health.

Understanding the complicated connection between these carotenoids and human health necessitates more study, making continuous research vital to determining their entire spectrum of advantages and uses.

This increasing corpus of scientific knowledge emphasizes the necessity of ongoing research and underlines the potential for lutein and zeaxanthin to benefit human health in a variety of ways.

CHAPTER 9

Special Considerations

Lutein And Zeaxanthin In Pregnancy

Various nutrients, particularly those that promote eyesight and general health, are in higher need during pregnancy. Because lutein and zeaxanthin are important for eye health, they also play a role in prenatal development. According to research, these carotenoids may have a good influence on baby visual development, leading to improved eye health and maybe lowering the risk of some eye diseases later in life. As a result, maintaining appropriate consumption of these nutrients throughout pregnancy may assist the growing child.

Furthermore, maternal diet affects the concentration of these carotenoids in breast milk, which adds to the infant's intake and general eye health.

Pediatric Health

Lutein and zeaxanthin are also beneficial to children. These substances are essential for the development and maintenance of visual function, helping to avoid eye illnesses such as age-related macular degeneration (AMD), cataracts, and other vision-related difficulties. Encouraging the intake of carotenoid-rich foods throughout infancy may benefit long-term eye health.

Furthermore, some evidence shows that enough lutein and zeaxanthin consumption throughout infancy may benefit cognitive development and learning ability. However, further research is required to determine the specific processes and relationships.

Aging Population

Maintaining eye health becomes more important as people age. Lutein and zeaxanthin are important for the aging population because they protect against age-related eyesight deterioration. These carotenoids work as antioxidants, reducing oxidative stress in the eyes produced by light exposure and environmental factors.

Higher amounts of lutein and zeaxanthin in the diet have been demonstrated in studies to lessen the chance of developing age-related eye diseases such as AMD and cataracts. Furthermore, continuing study is looking at the possible cognitive advantages of these carotenoids in older persons, including their involvement in maintaining brain health and cognitive performance.

Finally, maintaining enough intake of lutein and zeaxanthin during various life phases, such as pregnancy, childhood, and as one age, has tremendous potential for supporting eye health, cognitive function, and general well-being. More thorough research, however, is required to properly appreciate the depth and breadth of their effects on these particular groups.

CHAPTER 10
Future Trends And Developments

Lutein and zeaxanthin, formerly recognized solely for their function in eye health, are now emerging as interesting areas of study with potential uses well beyond vision. The future of these carotenoids is bright, with continued research and creative innovations.

Emerging Research Areas

Innovative research is diving further into the complex features of lutein and zeaxanthin. Researchers are discovering their impact on areas other than eye health, including cognitive function. According to research, they can support cognitive functions, perhaps lowering the risk of age-related cognitive decline. This developing area of inquiry investigates how carotenoids may affect brain health and neurological illnesses, generating interest in novel therapies.

Furthermore, the continuing study is looking at the link between Lutein and Zeaxanthin and chronic disorders including cardiovascular disease, diabetes, and potentially some malignancies. Preliminary data suggest that they can reduce inflammation, oxidative stress, and cellular damage, hinting at a larger range of health advantages that have yet to be completely explored.

Innovations In Delivery Methods

Novel delivery strategies are being investigated as research improves to improve the bioavailability and absorption of lutein and zeaxanthin. Nano-encapsulation and liposomal technologies are used in formulations to improve their stability and absorption, possibly boosting their effectiveness in the body. These advancements have the potential to improve supplementing techniques by assuring appropriate consumption and usage of these essential substances.

Potential Applications Beyond Health

Lutein and Zeaxanthin have fascinating non-medical possibilities in addition to their significance in human health. Their antioxidant capabilities are being researched for culinary and cosmetic uses. Extracts are being investigated for their preservation properties in food items, while their skin-protective properties are gaining attention in cosmetics formulations, possibly giving natural alternatives to sun protection.

Furthermore, these carotenoids are being included in animal feed formulations, notably for poultry and aquaculture, to improve the nutritional quality of animal-derived products.

The future of Lutein and Zeaxanthin research is bright, with a growing knowledge of their numerous uses and potential advantages. However, like with any new topic, further study is needed to confirm these results and fully understand their ramifications.

These trends and improvements highlight Lutein and Zeaxanthin's revolutionary potential beyond traditional bounds, providing a look into a future in which these compounds might play crucial roles in health, industry, and numerous aspects of everyday life.

Conclusion

Exploring the domains of Lutein and Zeaxanthin reveals that these carotenoids have benefits that go beyond their reputation as vision-enhancing agents. These chemicals are significant not just for their structural functions inside the eye, but also for their diverse benefits to general health.

These carotenoids, which have a distinct chemical structure, may be found in a variety of foods, most notably dark leafy greens, fruits, and vegetables. They are distinguished from other carotenoids by their presence in the macula of the eye, where they operate as potent antioxidants, preventing oxidative damage caused by damaging light exposure.

Numerous variables impact lutein and zeaxanthin absorption and bioavailability. While supplements are available, the body frequently absorbs these substances better from natural food sources, underlining the need for a nutritious diet.

Lutein and Zeaxanthin have health advantages that go beyond eye health. Their antioxidant qualities contribute significantly to cardiovascular health by lowering the risk of certain heart diseases. Furthermore, these chemicals have promise benefits on skin health, providing protection against UV-induced damage and perhaps alleviating age-related skin disorders.

Understanding optimal food consumption is critical in avoiding deficiencies. Although no RDA exists, research shows that these carotenoids should be consumed at optimum amounts. Individuals at increased risk of deficiency include those who consume less vegetables and have specific medical disorders, emphasizing the need for dietary changes or supplementation.

Foods high in Lutein and Zeaxanthin are essential components of a healthy diet. Cooking and processing processes, on the other hand, might alter their composition, underlining the significance of conscious food preparation approaches to keep these vital nutrients.

Scientific study is still revealing the many advantages of lutein and zeaxanthin. Ongoing studies investigate their potential in a variety of health-related areas, sometimes igniting arguments and conflicts within the scientific community and emphasizing the need for more extensive study.

Pregnant women, children, and the elderly need special consideration when it comes to consuming

Lutein and Zeaxanthin. Studies are being conducted to investigate their effects during pregnancy, on juvenile health, and their possible function in preventing age-related visual problems in the elderly.

To summarize, the importance of Lutein and Zeaxanthin goes much beyond their recognized involvement in eye health. A diet high in these chemicals not only improves eyesight but also improves general health. While additional study is needed, including these carotenoids in daily meals seems to be a wise decision for improving health outcomes. Their potential health advantages in a variety of areas highlight the need to eat a diet rich in these essential nutrients for a healthy future.

THE END

55